SMOOTHIES AND JUICING RECIPE

for

OSTEOPOROSIS REVERSAL

NUTRITIOUS BLENDS TO PROMOTE
HEALTHY STRONG BONES

LAKEISHA   OWENS

Published in 2024

TABLE OF CONTENT

INTRODUCTION

Osteoporosis is a condition characterized by weakened bones, which increases the risk of fractures and can significantly impact one's quality of life. However, with the right dietary choices, it is possible to enhance bone health, improve overall well-being, and mitigate some of the condition's effects.

This book is born out of a deep understanding of the crucial role that nutrition plays in bone health. It is grounded in the latest nutritional science and tailored specifically to meet the needs of those seeking to strengthen their bones and prevent further deterioration. Our recipes are more than just a collection, they are a fusion of flavor, health, and science, carefully curated to provide essential nutrients like calcium, vitamin D, magnesium, and potassium, which are vital for bone health.

Our mission is to empower you with knowledge and tools in the form of delicious, nutrient-packed smoothies and juices. Each recipe has been crafted with the goal of making it easier for you to incorporate bone-strengthening nutrients into your daily diet. We believe that managing osteoporosis and improving your bone health does not have to be a daunting task. By integrating these recipes into your routine, you can enjoy a variety of flavors while nourishing your body in a way that supports bone density and reduces the risk of fractures.

"Smoothies and Juicing Recipes for Osteoporosis" is more than just a recipe book; it's a companion on your journey to improved bone health. Through each page, we aim to inspire and guide you towards a lifestyle that not only addresses the needs of your bones but also delights your senses and enhances your overall well-being. Here's to a stronger, healthier you, one sip at a time.

JUICE RECIPE

JUICE RECIPE

Kale and Apple Bone Booster

Ingredients:

4 kale leaves

2 green apples, cored

1 cucumber

1/2 lemon, peeled

Instructions:

Wash all ingredients thoroughly.

Juice the kale, apples, cucumber, and lemon through a juicer.

Stir and serve immediately.

Nutritional Value:

Rich in calcium, vitamin C, and antioxidants.

Kale provides vitamin K, essential for bone health.

Calcium-Rich Orange Dream

Ingredients:

4 oranges, peeled

1/2 cup almonds, soaked overnight

2 carrots

Instructions:

Juice the oranges and carrots.

Blend the juice with soaked almonds until smooth.

Serve for a boost of calcium and vitamin C.

Nutritional Value:

Oranges and carrots provide vitamin C

Almonds add calcium and healthy fats.

Beetroot and Berry Magnesium Mix

Ingredients:

2 beetroots, peeled

1 cup strawberries

1 apple, cored

1/2-inch ginger

Instructions:

Juice the beetroots, strawberries, apple, and ginger.

Stir well and serve chilled.

Nutritional Value:

Beetroots and strawberries are rich in magnesium, which is

crucial for bone health.

Ginger adds anti-inflammatory properties.

Spinach and Carrot Calcium Juice

Ingredients:

3 cups spinach

3 carrots

1 apple, cored

Instructions:

Thoroughly wash the spinach, carrots, and apple.

Juice all ingredients and stir well.

Serve immediately to maximize nutrient intake.

Nutritional Value:

Spinach is high in calcium and magnesium

Carrots and apples add beta-carotene and fiber.

Tropical Turmeric Tonic

Ingredients:

1 cup pineapple chunks

1 mango, peeled and pitted

1/2-inch turmeric root

1 lime, peeled

Instructions:

Juice the pineapple, mango, turmeric, and lime.

Mix well and enjoy this anti-inflammatory and bone-strengthening drink.

Nutritional Value:

Pineapple and mango provide vitamin C and other antioxidants.

Turmeric is known for its anti-inflammatory properties.

Green Cucumber Cooler

Ingredients:

2 cucumbers

4 celery stalks

1/2 green apple, cored

1/4 cup parsley

Instructions:

Juice the cucumbers, celery, apple, and parsley.

Stir well and serve immediately for a refreshing and nutrient-rich juice.

Nutritional Value:

Cucumbers and celery are hydrating

Parsley and green apple offer vitamins and minerals supportive of bone health.

Watermelon and Strawberry Limeade

Ingredients:

2 cups watermelon cubes

1 cup strawberries

Juice of 1 lime

Instructions:

Blend watermelon, strawberries, and lime juice until smooth.

Strain if desired and serve immediately.

Nutritional Value:

Watermelon and strawberries provide hydration and antioxidants.

Lime adds vitamin C, enhancing iron absorption.

Pear and Ginger Bone Strengthener

Ingredients:

2 pears, cored – 348 grams

1/2-inch ginger – 2.5 grams

1 cucumber – 301 grams

Instructions:

Juice the pears, ginger, and cucumber.

Mix thoroughly and serve to enjoy its bone-supporting benefits.

Nutritional Value:

Pears offer boron and vitamin C, which are important for bone health.

Ginger contributes anti-inflammatory effects.

Broccoli and Apple Immune Boost

Ingredients:

1 cup broccoli florets

2 green apples, cored

1/2 lemon, peeled

Instructions:

Juice the broccoli, apples, and lemon.

Stir the juice well and serve immediately.

Nutritional Value:

Broccoli is rich in calcium and vitamin C

Apples add dietary fiber and antioxidants.

Sweet Potato Wellness Juice

Ingredients:

1 medium sweet potato, peeled

2 oranges, peeled

1 carrot

Instructions:

Juice the sweet potato, oranges, and carrot.

Mix well and enjoy this unique, nutrient-dense drink.

Nutritional Value:

Sweet potatoes provide beta-carotene and potassium.

Oranges add vitamin C, supporting collagen production for

bone and joint health.

Kale Pineapple Hydrator

Ingredients:

2 cups kale leaves

1 cup pineapple chunks

1 cucumber

1/2 lime, peeled

Instructions:

Juice all the ingredients together.

Stir well and serve this hydrating and bone-healthy juice.

Nutritional Value:

Kale is a powerhouse of calcium and antioxidants.

Pineapple adds bromelain, which may benefit bone health

and reduce inflammation.

Almond Milk and Berry Antioxidant Juice

Ingredients:

1 cup mixed berries (blueberries, raspberries, strawberries)

2 cups almond milk

1 banana

Instructions:

Blend the berries, almond milk, and banana until smooth.

Serve this creamy, antioxidant-rich juice for a delicious bone health boost.

Nutritional Value:

Berries are high in antioxidants and vitamin C, supporting overall health.

Almond milk provides a dairy-free calcium source

Bananas add potassium and vitamin B6.

Celery and Green Apple Digestive Aid

Ingredients:

4 celery stalks

2 green apples, cored

1 inch ginger root

1/2 lemon, peeled

Instructions:

Juice the celery, green apples, ginger, and lemon.

Stir well and serve to aid digestion and support bone health.

Nutritional Value:

Celery and apples are hydrating and provide essential nutrients.

Ginger and lemon boost digestion and offer anti-inflammatory benefits.

Carrot and Turmeric Anti-Inflammatory Juice

Ingredients:

5 carrots

1/2-inch turmeric root

1 orange, peeled

1/2 lemon, peeled

Instructions:

Juice the carrots, turmeric, orange, and lemon.

Mix well and enjoy the anti-inflammatory and bone-strengthening properties.

Nutritional Value:

Carrots are rich in beta-carotene and vitamin K.

Turmeric is known for its curcumin content, which supports bone density and reduces inflammation.

Spinach, Cucumber, and Mint Refresh

Ingredients:

3 cups spinach

1 cucumber

1/2 cup mint leaves

2 kiwis, peeled

Instructions:

Juice the spinach, cucumber, mint, and kiwis.

Stir well and serve this refreshing and nutrient-packed juice.

Nutritional Value:

Spinach provides iron and calcium, essential for bone health.

Cucumber and mint offer hydration and digestive benefits

Kiwi brings vitamin C and K, crucial for bone and overall

health.

SMOOTHIE RECIPE

SMOOTHIE RECIPE

Calcium Powerhouse Smoothie

Ingredients:

2 cups fortified almond milk (rich in calcium and vitamin D)

1 cup kale, chopped

2 medium bananas

4 tablespoons almond butter

2 teaspoons chia seeds

Instructions:

Combine all ingredients in a blender.

Blend on high until smooth and creamy.

Serve immediately for best taste and nutrient retention.

Nutritional Value:

Rich in calcium, vitamin D, potassium, and healthy fats from almond butter.

Chia seeds add omega-3 fatty acids and additional calcium.

Berry Bone Booster

Ingredients:

1 cup Greek yogurt (high in calcium)

1 cup frozen mixed berries (strawberries, blueberries, raspberries)

1 cup spinach leaves

1 cup orange juice (fortified with calcium and vitamin D)

1 tablespoon flaxseed meal

Instructions:

Add all ingredients to a blender.

Blend until smooth.

Enjoy immediately, ensuring maximum nutrient preservation.

Nutritional Value:

Offers a good dose of calcium, antioxidants, vitamin C, and vitamin D.

Flaxseed meal contributes to omega-3 fatty acids and fiber.

Mango Ginger Magic

Ingredients:

2 cups frozen mango chunks

2 cups carrot juice (natural source of calcium)

1 tablespoon grated ginger

1 banana

1 tablespoon turmeric powder

Instructions:

Place all ingredients in a blender.

Puree until smooth.

Serve this vibrant smoothie immediately for a refreshing treat.

Nutritional Value:

Packed with vitamin A from carrot juice and mango, calcium, and anti-inflammatory properties from ginger and turmeric.

Peachy Almond Delight

Ingredients:

2 ripe peaches, sliced

2 cups spinach

2 cups almond milk (calcium-fortified)

4 tablespoons almond butter

1 teaspoon vanilla extract

Instructions:

Combine peaches, spinach, almond milk, almond butter, and

vanilla extract in a blender.

Blend until smooth.

Serve chilled for a refreshing, nutrient-rich drink.

Nutritional Value:

A great source of calcium, vitamin E from almond butter,

and vitamin C from peaches.

Spinach adds iron and fiber.

Sweet Potato Pie Smoothie

Ingredients:

1 medium sweet potato, cooked and cooled

2 cups almond milk (calcium-fortified)

1 banana

1 teaspoon cinnamon

1/2 teaspoon nutmeg

2 tablespoons maple syrup

Instructions:

Add all ingredients into a blender.

Blend until smooth and well combined.

Serve immediately for a sweet and nutritious treat.

Nutritional Value:

High in calcium, beta-carotene (from sweet potato), and spices that support metabolic health.

Avocado Greens Smoothie

Ingredients:

1 ripe avocado

2 cups kale leaves

2 cups fortified soy milk

2 tablespoons hemp seeds

1 lemon, juiced

Instructions:

Place avocado, kale, soy milk, hemp seeds, and lemon juice

in a blender.

Blend until creamy.

Enjoy this creamy, nutritious blend immediately.

Nutritional Value:

Rich in healthy fats, calcium, vitamin K, and protein.

Hemp seeds add omega-3s and additional protein.

Blueberry Walnut Wonder

Ingredients:

2 cups blueberries (fresh or frozen)

2 bananas

2 cups spinach

2 cups rice milk (calcium-fortified)

4 tablespoons walnuts

Instructions:

Combine blueberries, bananas, spinach, rice milk, and walnuts in a blender.

Blend until smooth.

Serve this antioxidant-rich smoothie promptly.

Nutritional Value:

Provides omega-3 fatty acids from walnuts, antioxidants from blueberries, calcium, and vitamin D from rice milk.

Cinnamon Roll Smoothie

Ingredients:

2 cups Greek yogurt (high in calcium)

2 bananas

2 teaspoons cinnamon

4 tablespoons oats

1 cup almond milk (calcium-fortified)

2 tablespoons honey

Instructions:

Add all ingredients to a blender.

Blend until smooth and creamy.

Serve immediately, garnished with a sprinkle of cinnamon if desired.

Nutritional Value:

Loaded with calcium, probiotics from Greek yogurt, and heart-healthy oats.

Cinnamon adds anti-inflammatory properties.

Tropical Turmeric Smoothie

Ingredients:

2 cups coconut water

2 cups frozen pineapple chunks

1 mango, peeled and diced

1 tablespoon turmeric

1 teaspoon ginger, grated

Instructions:

Combine coconut water, pineapple, mango, turmeric, and ginger in a blender.

Blend until smooth.

Enjoy the immune-boosting and anti-inflammatory benefits of this smoothie.

Nutritional Value:

Excellent source of hydration from coconut water

Vitamin C from tropical fruits

The anti-inflammatory benefits of turmeric and ginger.

Green Tea Zen Smoothie

Ingredients:

2 cups brewed green tea, cooled

2 cups spinach leaves

1 avocado

2 teaspoons honey

1 inch ginger, grated

Instructions:

Place green tea, spinach, avocado, honey, and ginger in a blender.

Blend until smooth.

Serve this soothing smoothie for a calm start to your day or a relaxing afternoon treat.

Nutritional Value:

Green tea provides antioxidants and a gentle caffeine boost

While avocado offers healthy fats and fiber.

Spinach is a great source of calcium and iron

Ginger adds digestive and anti-inflammatory benefits.

Protein Punch Smoothie

Ingredients:

2 cups fortified oat milk

2 tablespoons peanut butter

1 banana

2 scoops protein powder (choose a brand fortified with calcium and vitamin D)

1 tablespoon cocoa powder

Instructions:

Combine oat milk, peanut butter, banana, protein powder, and cocoa powder in a blender.

Blend until smooth.

Enjoy this high-protein, nutrient-dense smoothie, perfect for post-workout recovery.

Nutritional Value:

High in protein, calcium, and potassium.

The peanut butter and banana add a comforting flavor, while the cocoa powder provides antioxidants.

Fig and Date Delight

Ingredients:

6 dried figs, soaked in water for 1 hour

4 dates, pitted and soaked

2 cups almond milk (calcium-fortified)

1 teaspoon cinnamon

2 tablespoons chia seeds

Instructions:

Drain figs and dates and add them to the blender with almond milk, cinnamon, and chia seeds.

Blend until smooth.

Serve this naturally sweet and nutrient-packed smoothie immediately.

Nutritional Value:

Figs and dates are rich in calcium and magnesium, essential for bone health.

Chia seeds add omega-3 fatty acids and fiber.

Avocado Berry Bliss

Ingredients:

1 avocado

2 cups mixed berries (strawberries, blueberries, raspberries)

2 cups spinach

2 cups coconut milk (calcium-fortified)

1 tablespoon honey (optional)

Instructions:

Place avocado, mixed berries, spinach, coconut milk, and

honey (if using) into a blender.

Blend until creamy and smooth.

Serve this creamy, antioxidant-rich smoothie to nourish your

body and bones.

Nutritional Value:

Rich in healthy fats from avocado

Calcium from coconut milk

A variety of vitamins and antioxidants from berries and

spinach.

Pumpkin Seed Power Smoothie

Ingredients:

2 cups soy milk (calcium and vitamin D fortified)

1/2 cup pumpkin seeds (soaked overnight)

2 bananas

1 teaspoon vanilla extract

1 tablespoon maple syrup

1/2 teaspoon cinnamon

Instructions:

Blend soy milk, soaked pumpkin seeds, bananas, vanilla extract, maple syrup, and cinnamon until smooth.

Serve this nutrient-dense smoothie, ideal for a healthy start to your day.

Nutritional Value:

Pumpkin seeds are a good source of magnesium, zinc, and healthy fats.

Soy milk provides calcium and vitamin D.

Bananas add potassium and natural sweetness.

Kiwi Lime Refresher

Ingredients:

4 kiwis, peeled and sliced

2 cups kale

2 cups water or coconut water

Juice of 2 limes

2 tablespoons honey

Instructions:

Add kiwis, kale, water/coconut water, lime juice, and honey to a blender.

Blend until smooth and refreshing.

Serve this vitamin C-packed smoothie to support immune function and bone health.

Nutritional Value:

Kiwis and kale provide a high dose of vitamin C and calcium.

Lime juice adds a refreshing zest and aids in the absorption of iron from the kale

Honey brings natural sweetness and energy.

CONCLUSION

The journey to improved bone health is not just about what we remove from our diets but what we choose to include. Through these recipes, we've seen how incorporating a wide array of fruits, vegetables, nuts, seeds, and fortified ingredients can not only enhance our nutritional intake but also bring joy and diversity to our meals. It's a testament to the fact that a diet aimed at combating osteoporosis doesn't have to be restrictive or bland but can be full of flavor and color. This book has served as a guide, offering a collection of recipes designed to fortify your body with essential nutrients crucial for bone density and strength.

Each recipe within these pages has been crafted with care, emphasizing the importance of calcium, vitamin D, magnesium, and other bone-beneficial nutrients. From the leafy greens of the Alkalizing Green Goddess Juice to the protein-packed delights of the Sesame Seed Banana Energy Smoothie, we've explored how delicious and varied your dietary choices can be, even within the specific needs of osteoporosis prevention and management.

As we close this book, let it not be the end of your exploration into the power of nutrition for bone health. Let it be a beginning, a foundation on which to build a lifestyle that embraces the richness of healthful foods. Experiment with these recipes, adjust them to your taste, and incorporate the principles they embody into your daily eating habits. Remember, the journey to stronger bones and a healthier body is a continuous one, and every nutrient-rich meal is a step in the right direction.

It is our hope that this book has empowered you with knowledge and inspired you with creativity. May your blender be your ally in health, and may each smoothie and juice you craft bring you closer to the vibrant wellness you deserve. Here's to your health, to your bones, and to a life lived with vitality and joy.

HAPPY BLENDING!!!!!!!!!!

DAILY MEAL PLANNER

DAILY
MEAL PLANNER

BREAKFAST

LUNCH

DINNER

SHOPPING LIST

DAILY
MEAL PLANNER

BREAKFAST

LUNCH

DINNER

SHOPPING LIST

DAILY
MEAL PLANNER

BREAKFAST

LUNCH

DINNER

SHOPPING LIST

DAILY
MEAL PLANNER

BREAKFAST

LUNCH

DINNER

SHOPPING LIST

DAILY
MEAL PLANNER

BREAKFAST

LUNCH

DINNER

SHOPPING LIST

DAILY
MEAL PLANNER

BREAKFAST

LUNCH

DINNER

SHOPPING LIST

DAILY
MEAL PLANNER

BREAKFAST

LUNCH

DINNER

SHOPPING LIST

DAILY
MEAL PLANNER

BREAKFAST

LUNCH

DINNER

SHOPPING LIST

DAILY
MEAL PLANNER

BREAKFAST

LUNCH

DINNER

SHOPPING LIST

DAILY
MEAL PLANNER

BREAKFAST

LUNCH

DINNER

SHOPPING LIST

DAILY
MEAL PLANNER

BREAKFAST

LUNCH

DINNER

SHOPPING LIST

DAILY
MEAL PLANNER

BREAKFAST

LUNCH

DINNER

SHOPPING LIST

DAILY
MEAL PLANNER

BREAKFAST

LUNCH

DINNER

SHOPPING LIST

DAILY
MEAL PLANNER

BREAKFAST

LUNCH

DINNER

SHOPPING LIST

DAILY
MEAL PLANNER

BREAKFAST

LUNCH

DINNER

SHOPPING LIST

DAILY
MEAL PLANNER

BREAKFAST

LUNCH

DINNER

SHOPPING LIST

DAILY
MEAL PLANNER

BREAKFAST

LUNCH

DINNER

SHOPPING LIST

DAILY
MEAL PLANNER

BREAKFAST

LUNCH

DINNER

SHOPPING LIST

DAILY
MEAL PLANNER

BREAKFAST

LUNCH

DINNER

SHOPPING LIST

DAILY
MEAL PLANNER

BREAKFAST

LUNCH

DINNER

SHOPPING LIST

DAILY
MEAL PLANNER

BREAKFAST

LUNCH

DINNER

SHOPPING LIST

DAILY
MEAL PLANNER

BREAKFAST

LUNCH

DINNER

SHOPPING LIST

DAILY
MEAL PLANNER

BREAKFAST

____

____

LUNCH

____

____

DINNER

____

____

SHOPPING LIST

DAILY
MEAL PLANNER

BREAKFAST

____

____

LUNCH

____

____

DINNER

____

____

SHOPPING LIST

DAILY
MEAL PLANNER

BREAKFAST

LUNCH

DINNER

SHOPPING LIST

DAILY
MEAL PLANNER

BREAKFAST

LUNCH

DINNER

SHOPPING LIST

DAILY
MEAL PLANNER

BREAKFAST

LUNCH

DINNER

SHOPPING LIST

DAILY
MEAL PLANNER

BREAKFAST

LUNCH

DINNER

SHOPPING LIST

DAILY
MEAL PLANNER

BREAKFAST

LUNCH

DINNER

SHOPPING LIST

DAILY
MEAL PLANNER

BREAKFAST

LUNCH

DINNER

SHOPPING LIST

DAILY
MEAL PLANNER

BREAKFAST

LUNCH

DINNER

SHOPPING LIST

DAILY
MEAL PLANNER

BREAKFAST

LUNCH

DINNER

SHOPPING LIST

9 798879 140217